WASH EM DOWN

Words by Tamika Mitchell-Wilcher

Pictures by Laney Fultz

Dowell HOUSE Publishing

Dowell House Publishing, LLC
2221 Hampstead Dr.
Columbus, OH 43229
www.dowellhousepublishing.com

ISBN: 979-8-9858200-1-0
Library of Congress #: 2022914308

Illustrations by Laney Fultz
Digital and Graphic Editing: Ashley E. Dowell
Photography by Tamika Mitchell-Wilcher

Printed in the United States of America

Disclaimer:

The words in this book are intended to be a comedic parody of the song **Walk Em Down by NLE Choppa. The words in this book have not been professionally recorded by Tamika Wilcher to the tune of "Walk Em Down" and are not being sold for profit as a musical single. For an example of how you can match the words with the tune "Walk Em Down," please visit Tamika Wilcher's social media channels for much "cleaner" and more educational versions of the original songs!

Sing along with the "Wash Em Down" book here: https://www.youtube.com/watch?v=69-pxB2htE0

Check out her other social media pages for more songs and content!

TikTok: @educatedauthor3
YouTube: Teacher T's World

**Walk Em Down ©2020 NLE Choppa Entertainment Inc., under exclusive license to Warner Records Inc.

Music Notes PNGs by Vecteezy..com

Dedication

I am eternally grateful for all of my "Cool Cats" that I have had the opportunity to stand before and lead. Thank you for being my inspiration and entering the classroom ready to learn each day. I love you all so very much!

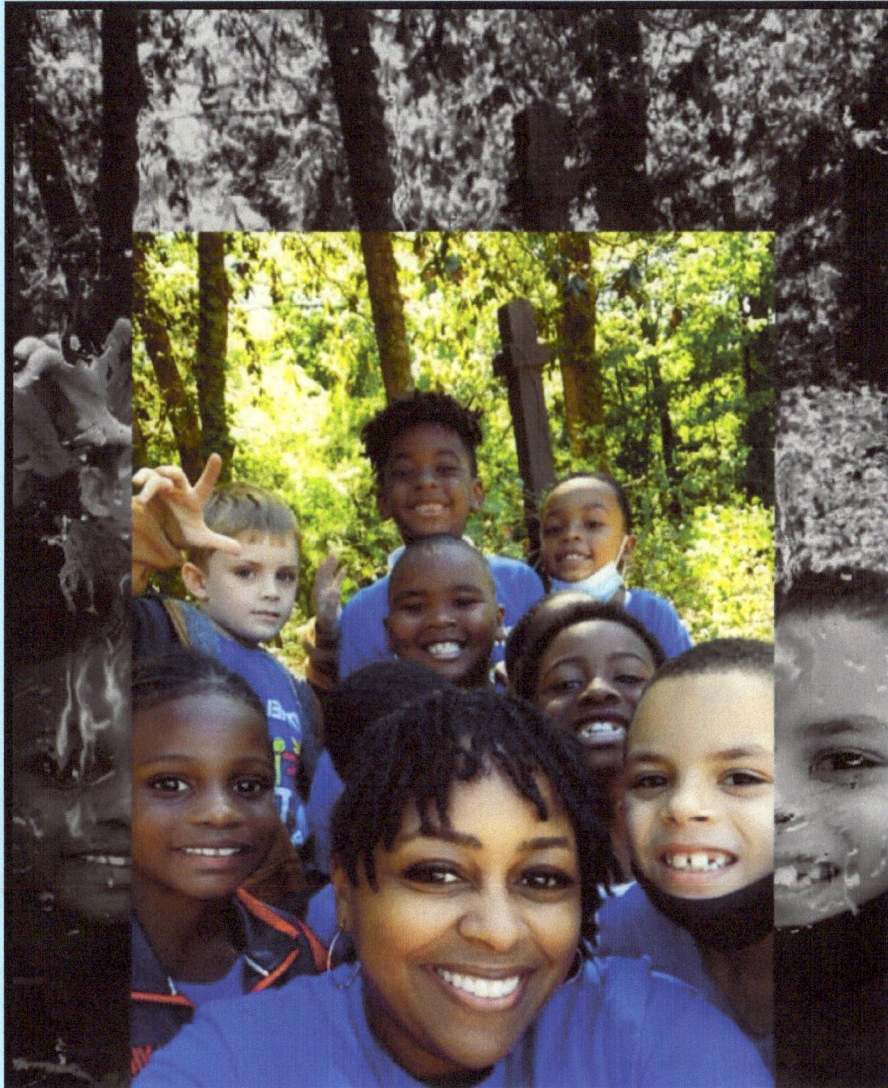

Posted in front of the sink.

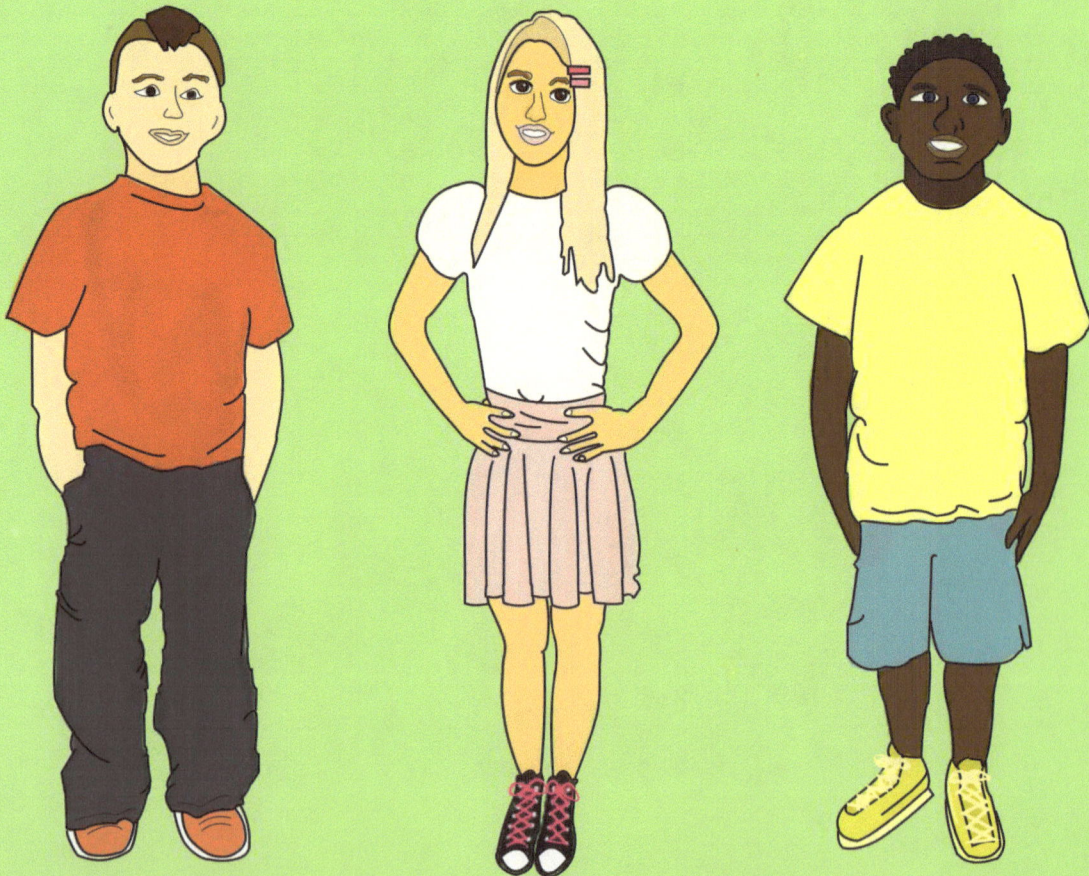

Getting ready to watch them germs go down!

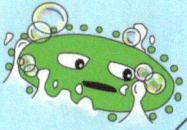

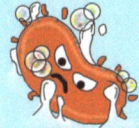

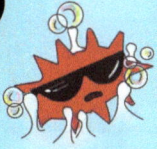

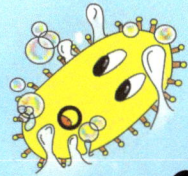

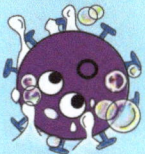

2

Turn on the tap
and apply the soap!

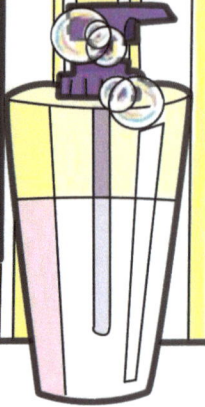

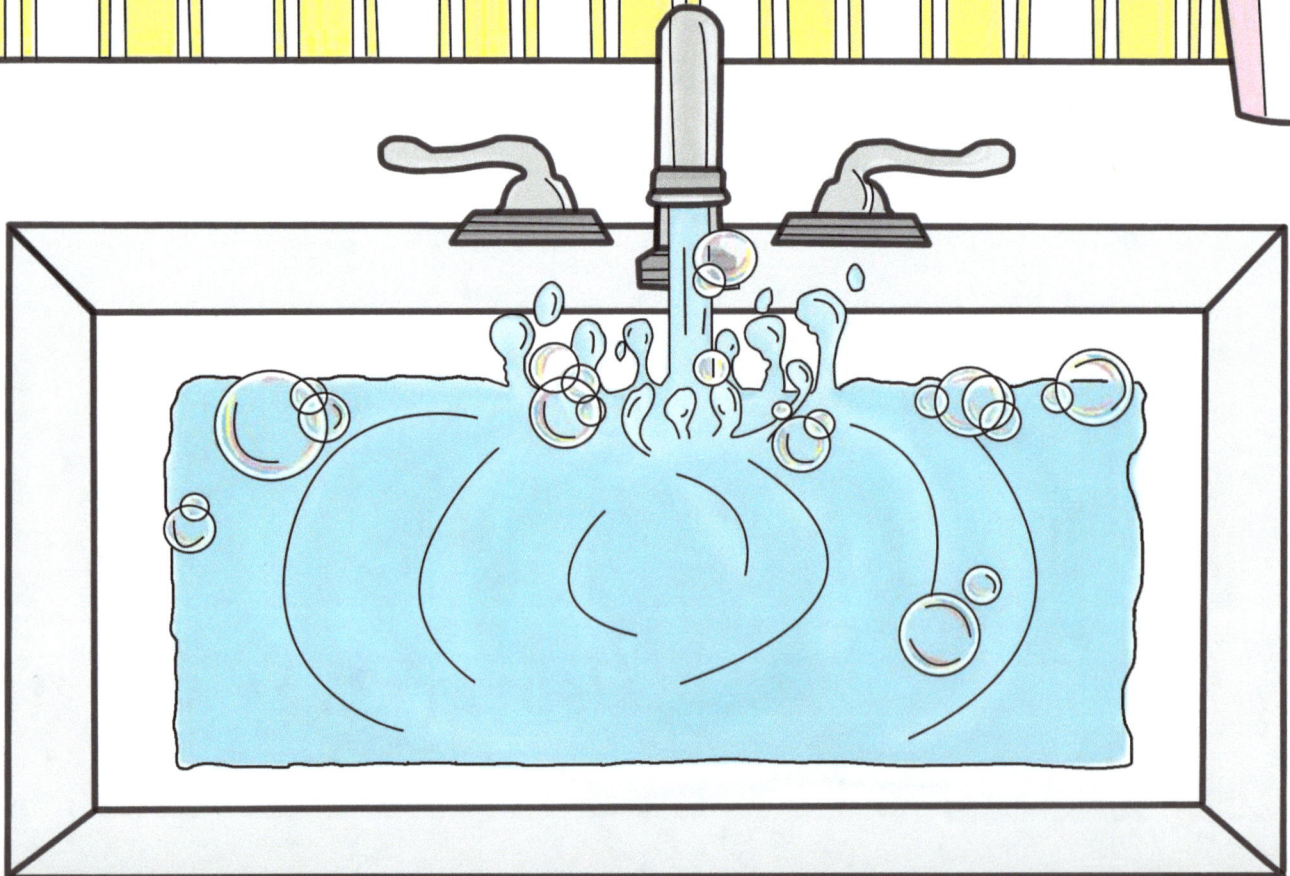

Then we make the hands go round and round.

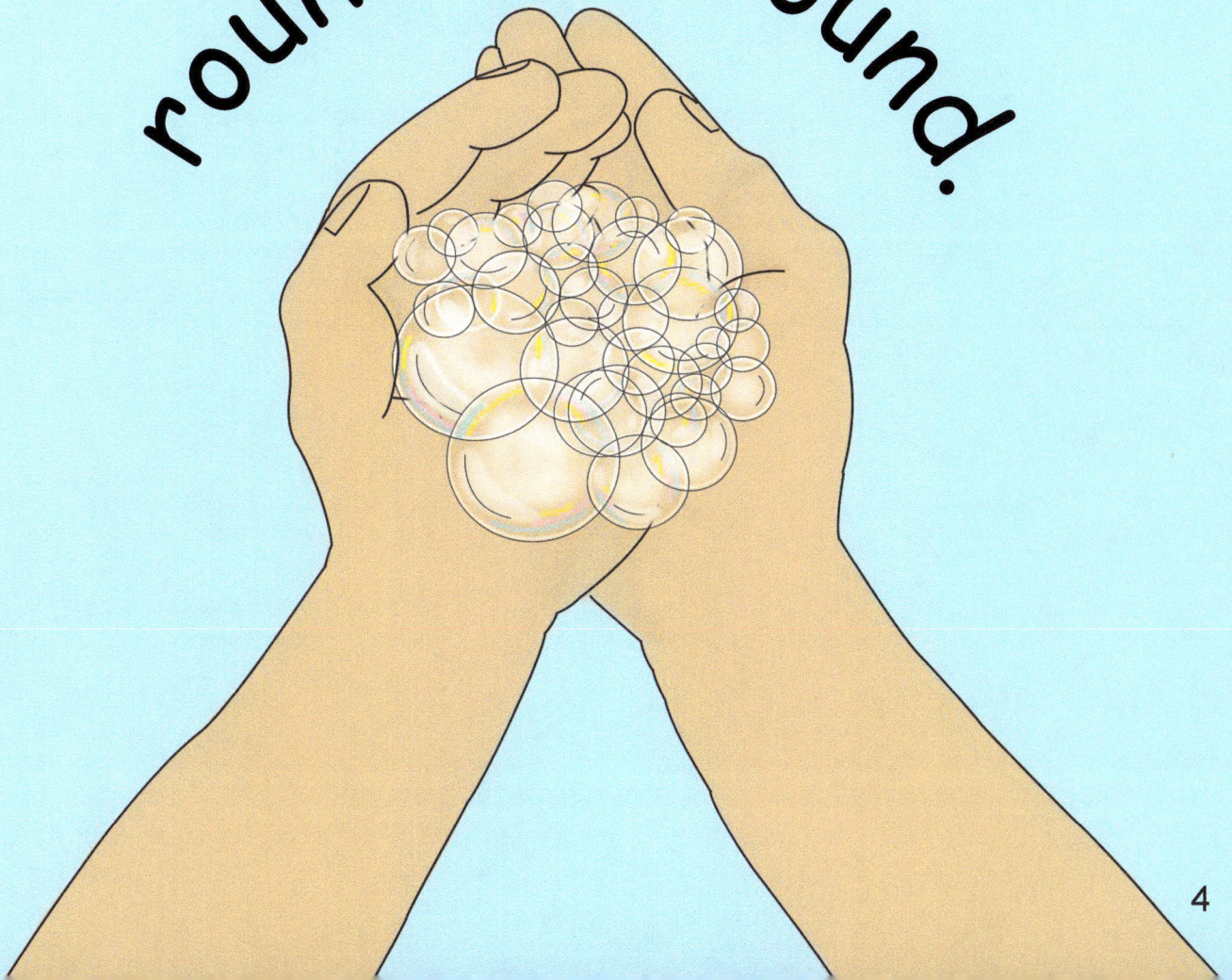

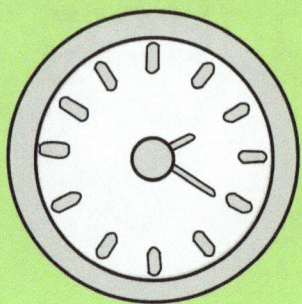

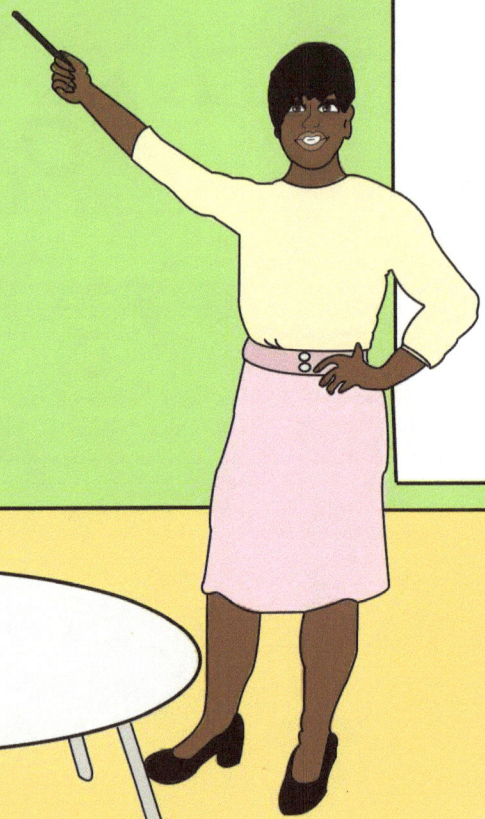

Teachers in the back with the clock.

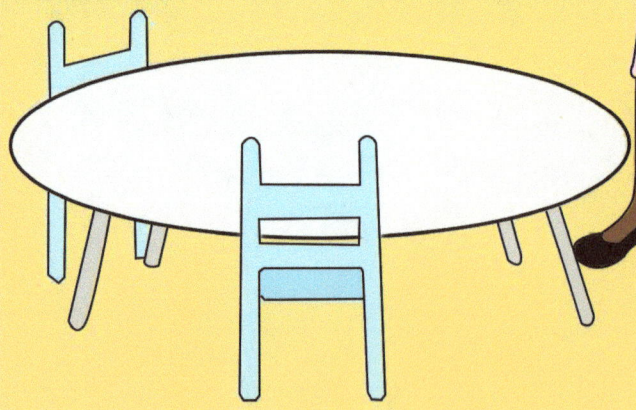

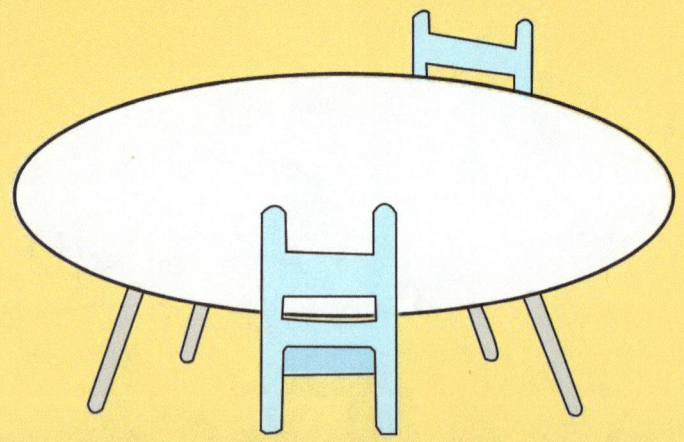

We got 20 seconds to make them germs go down.

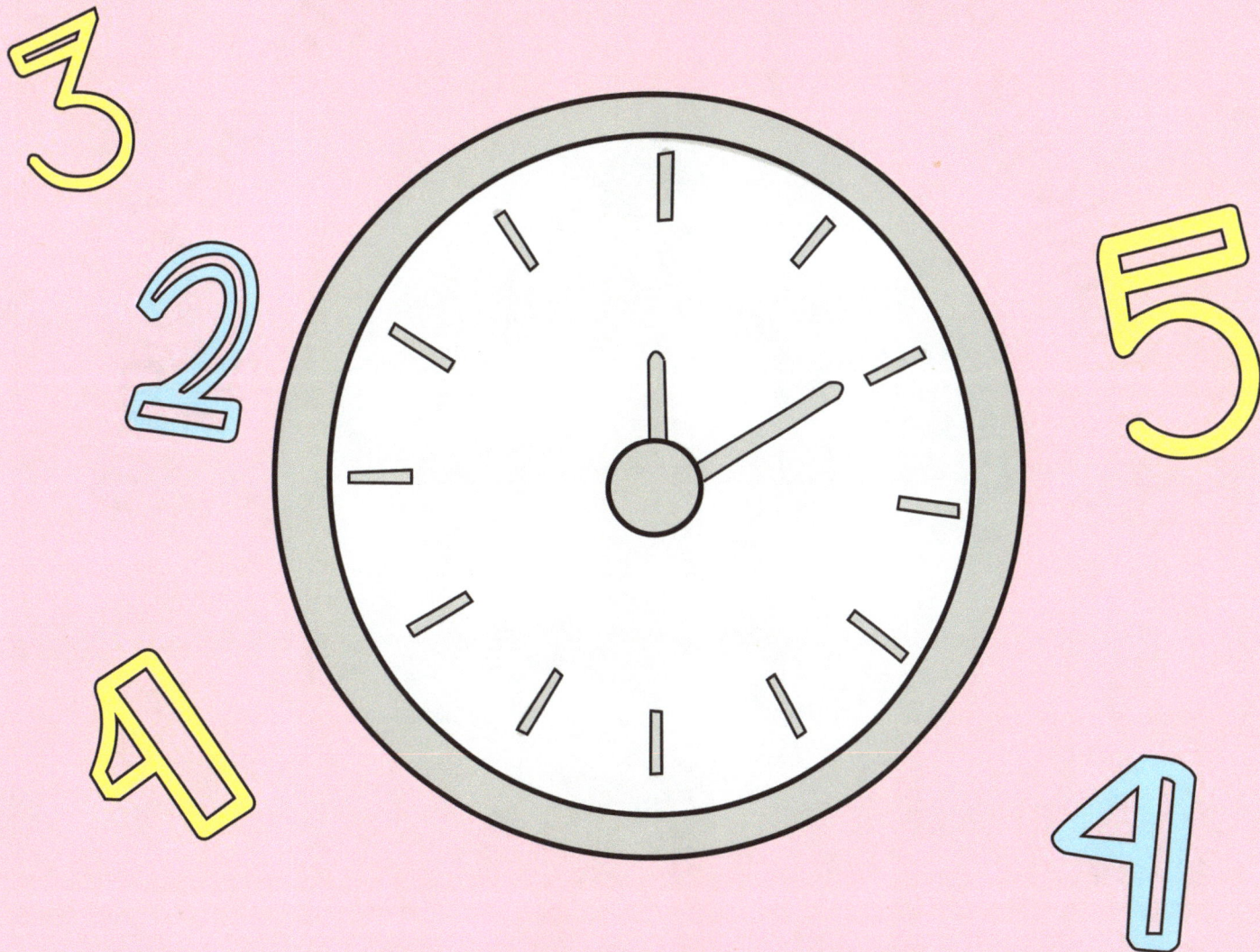

You think we hesitating 'cause she ain't playin'.

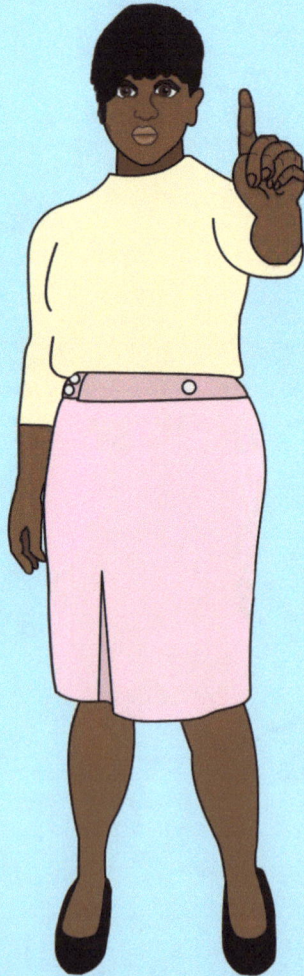

She **DON'T** like them germs and we can't let her down.

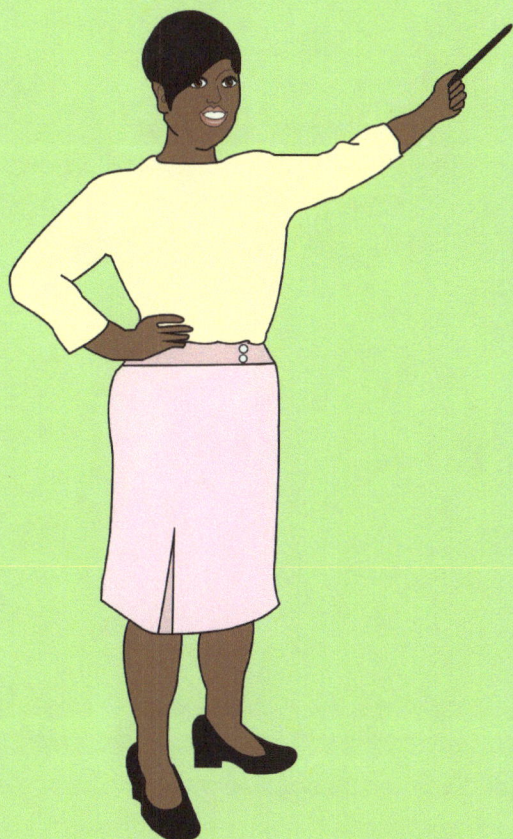

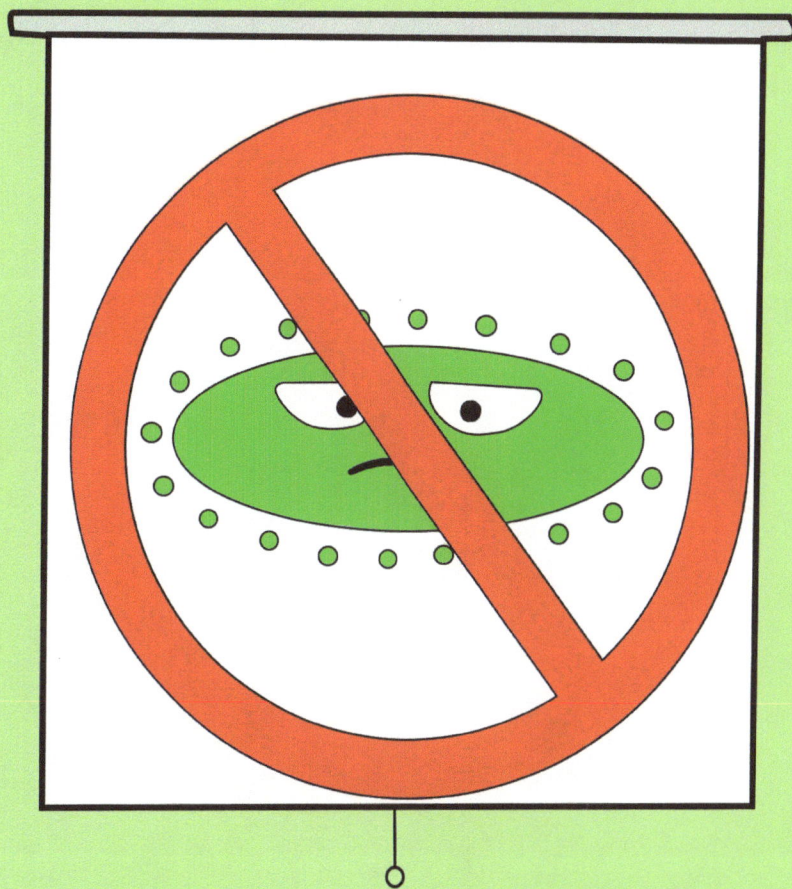

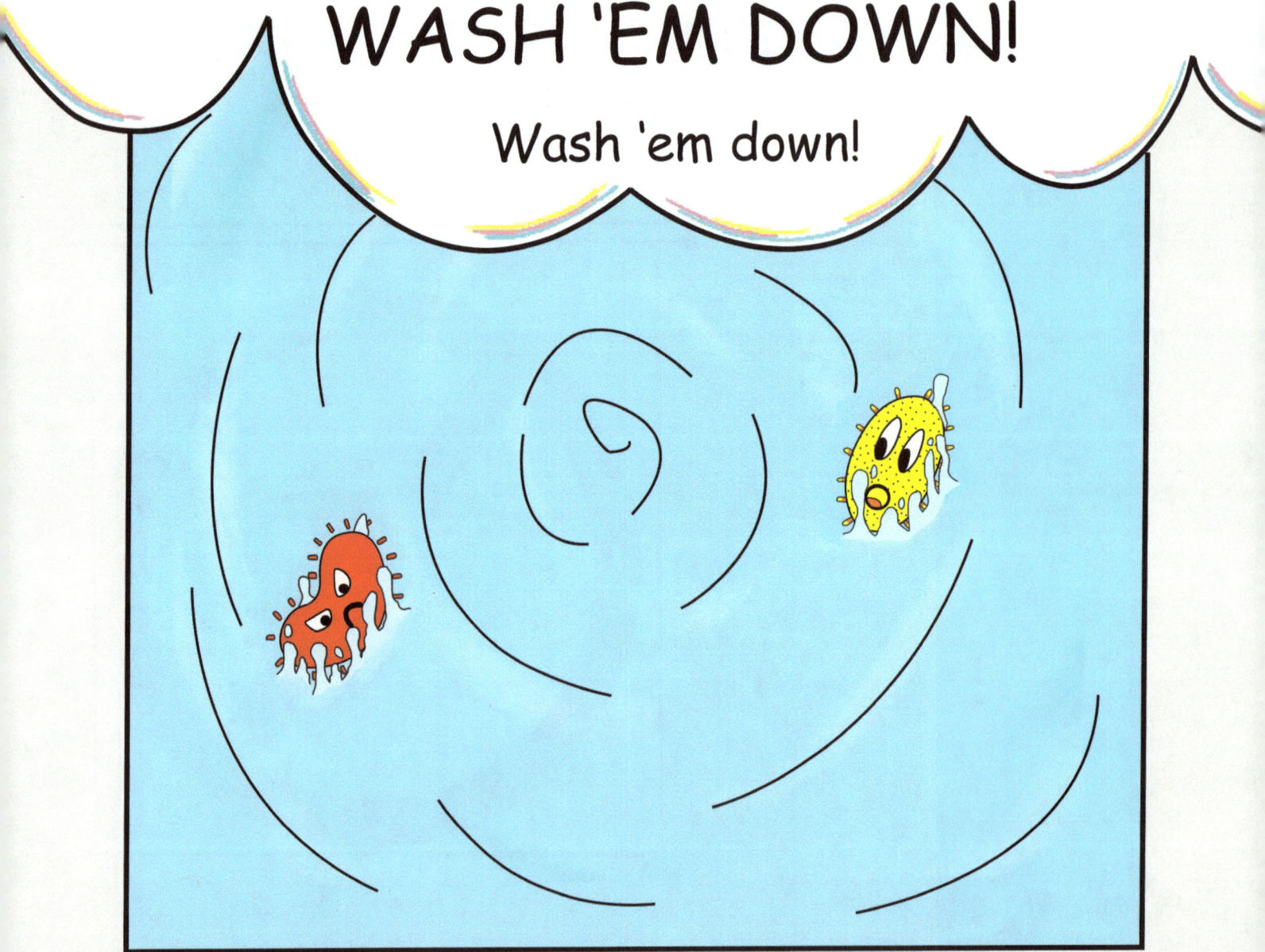

9

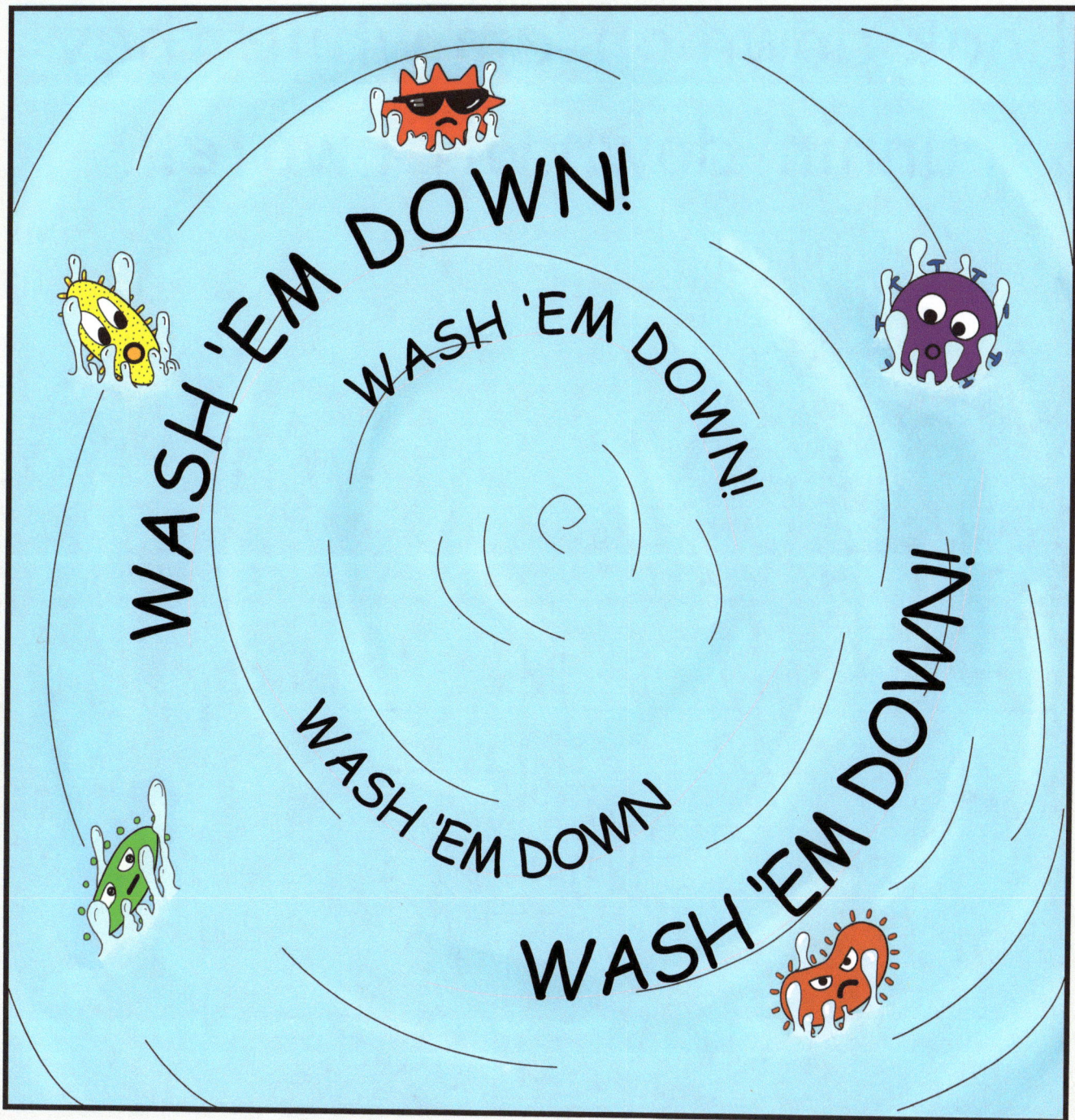

Look down on 'em while they runnin' down with water.

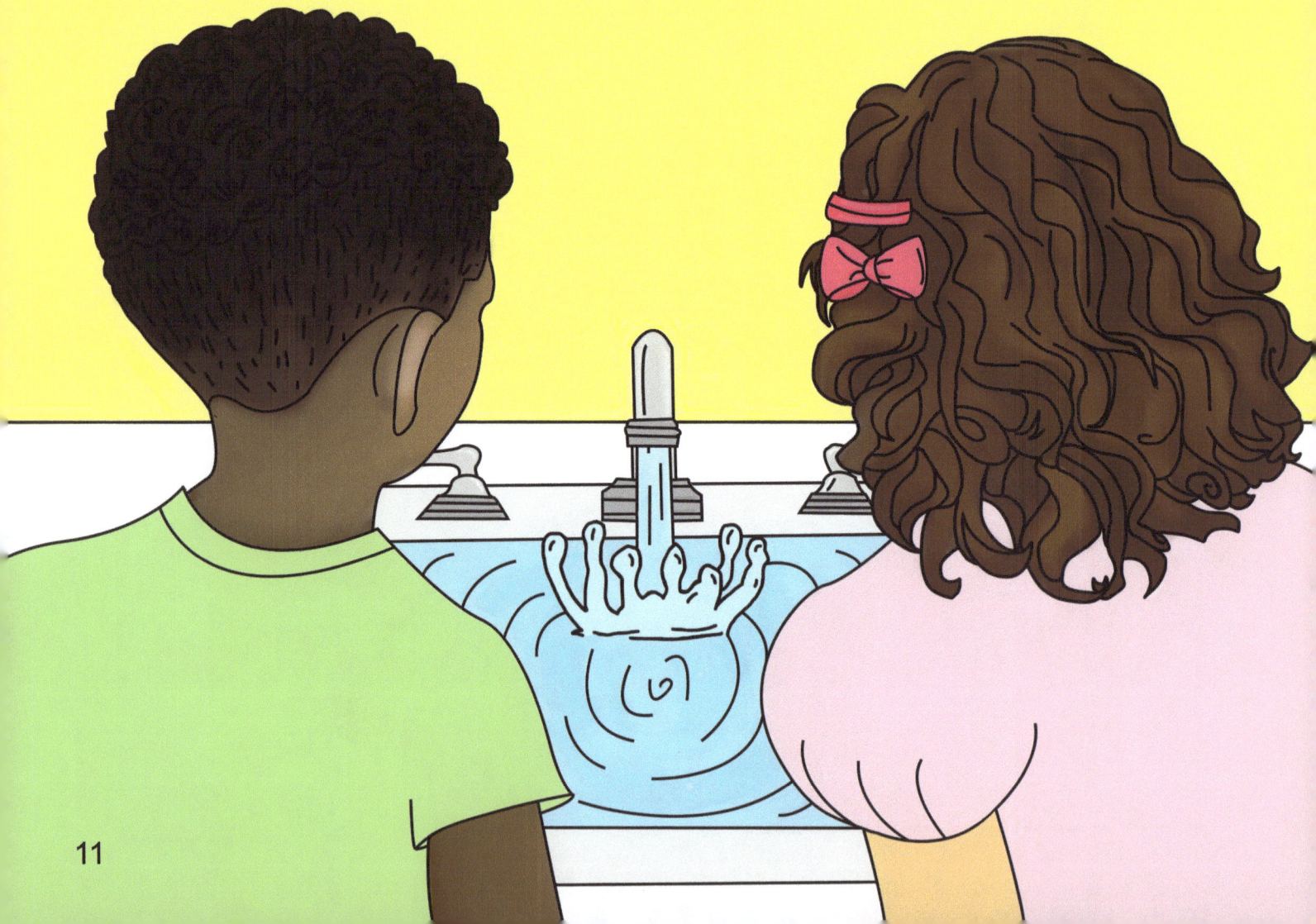

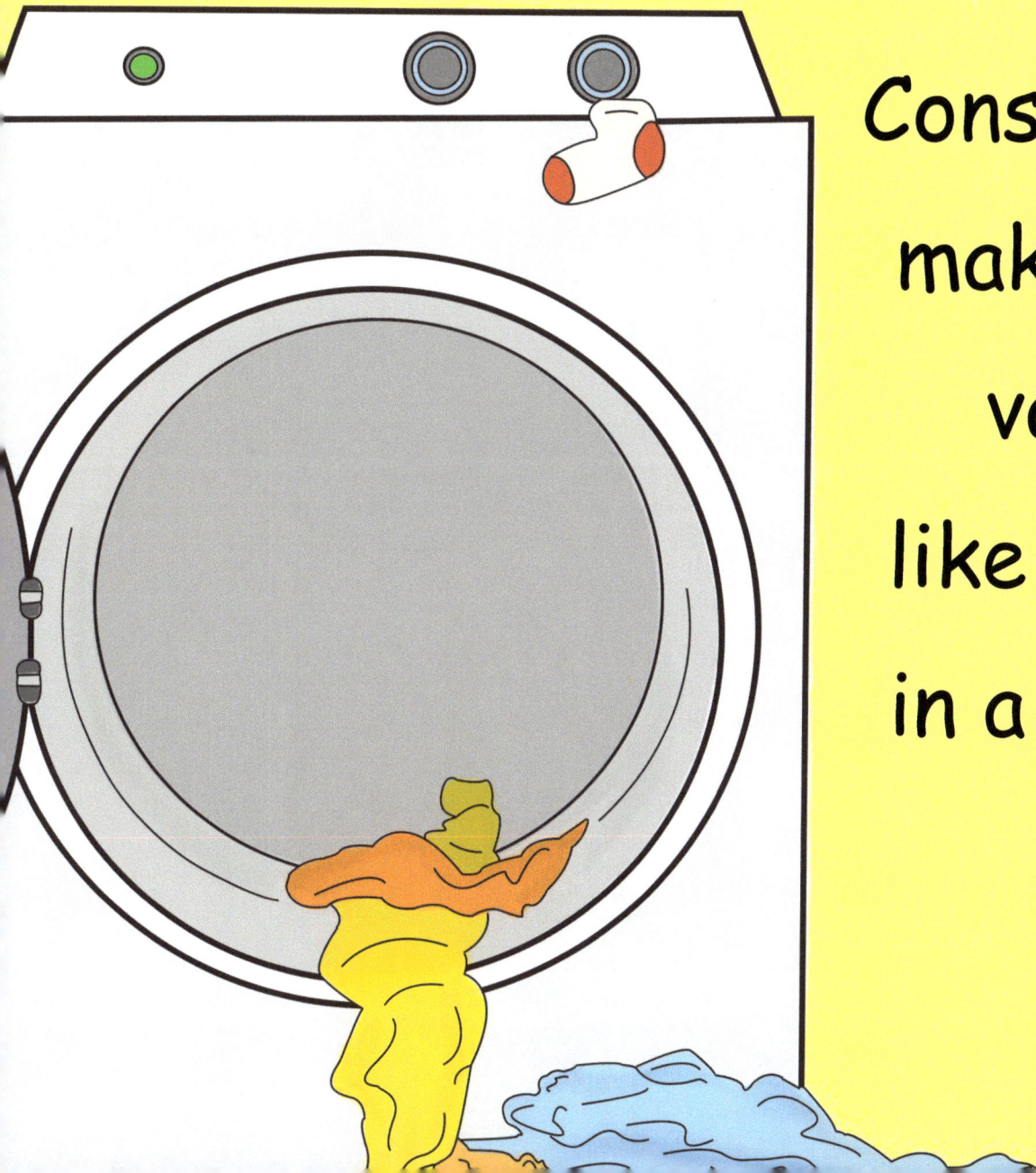

Consistency
makes 'em
vanish
like a sock
in a dryer.

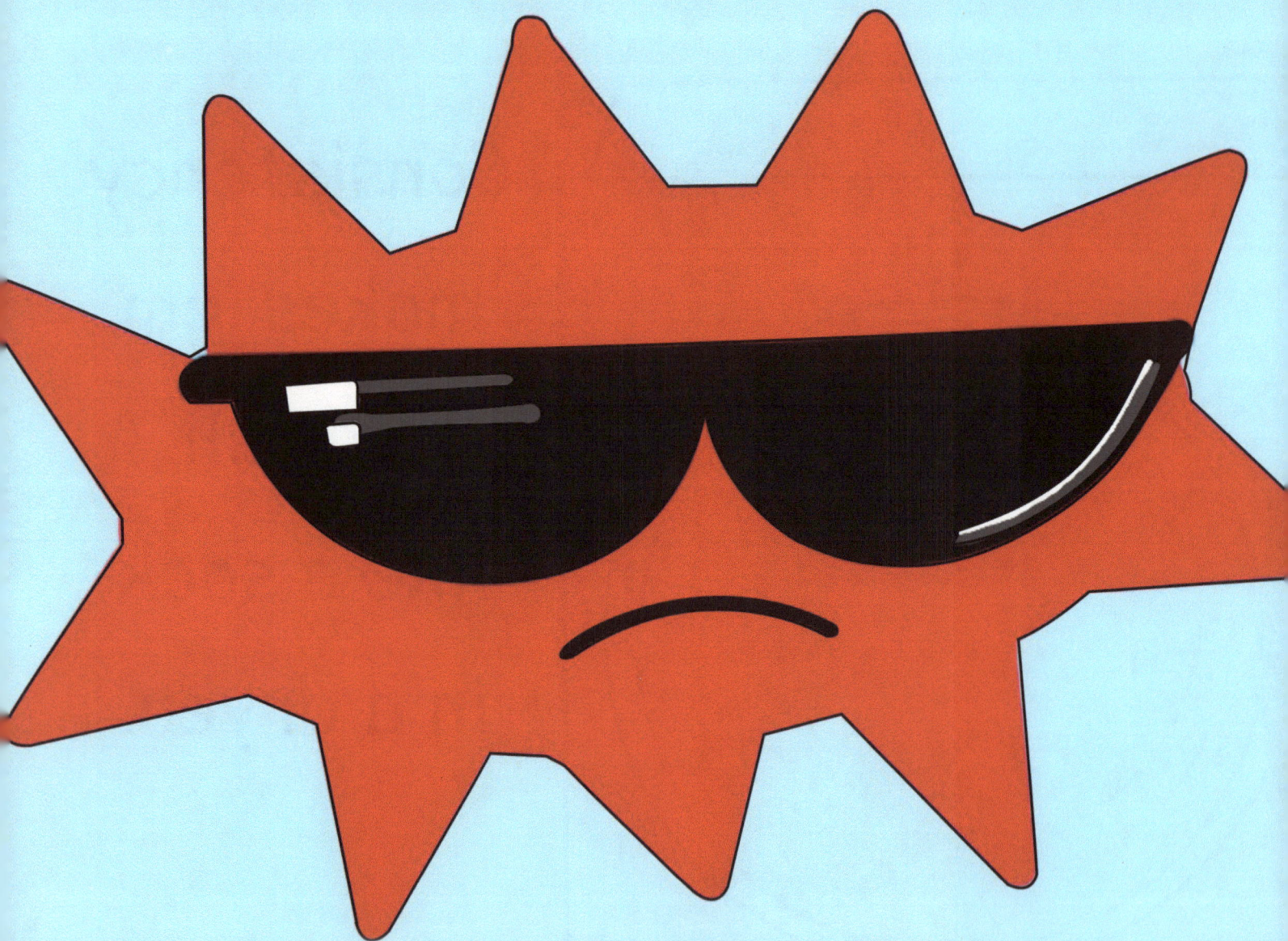

We make them hands go round and round like it's good karma.

14

They look really clean now,
but I wanna wash 'em.

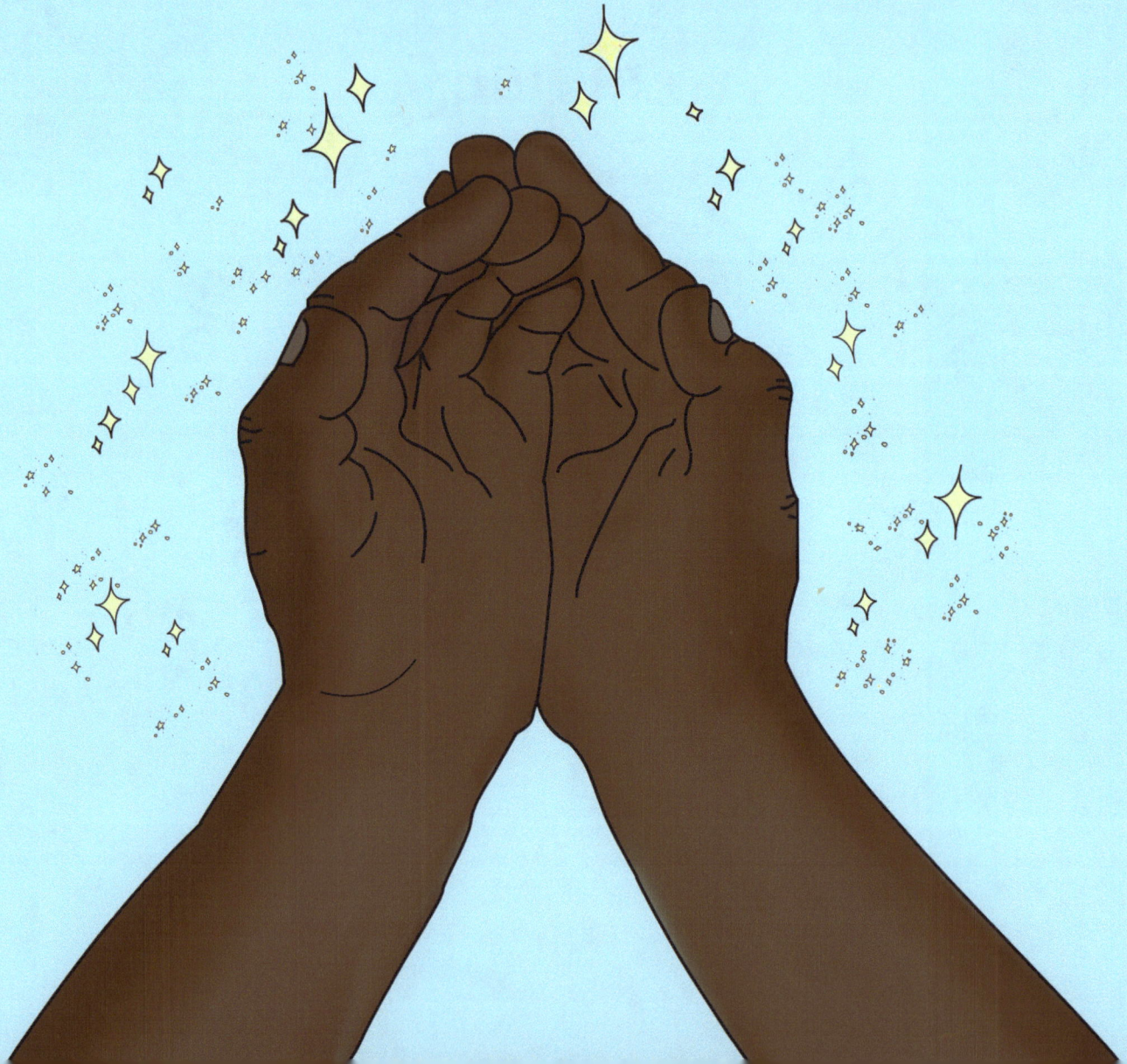

I know I can't see them germs, but I want to stalk 'em.

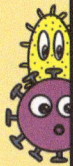

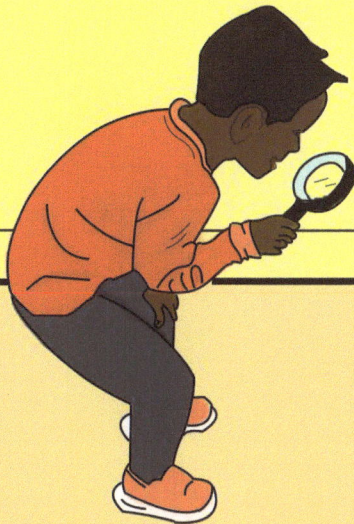

Caution tape round the sink.
I had to destroy 'em!

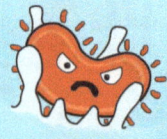
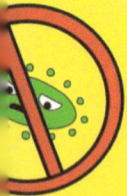
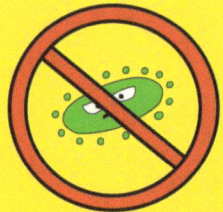
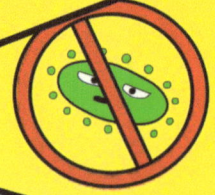
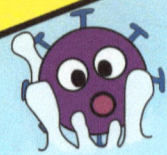

CAUTION

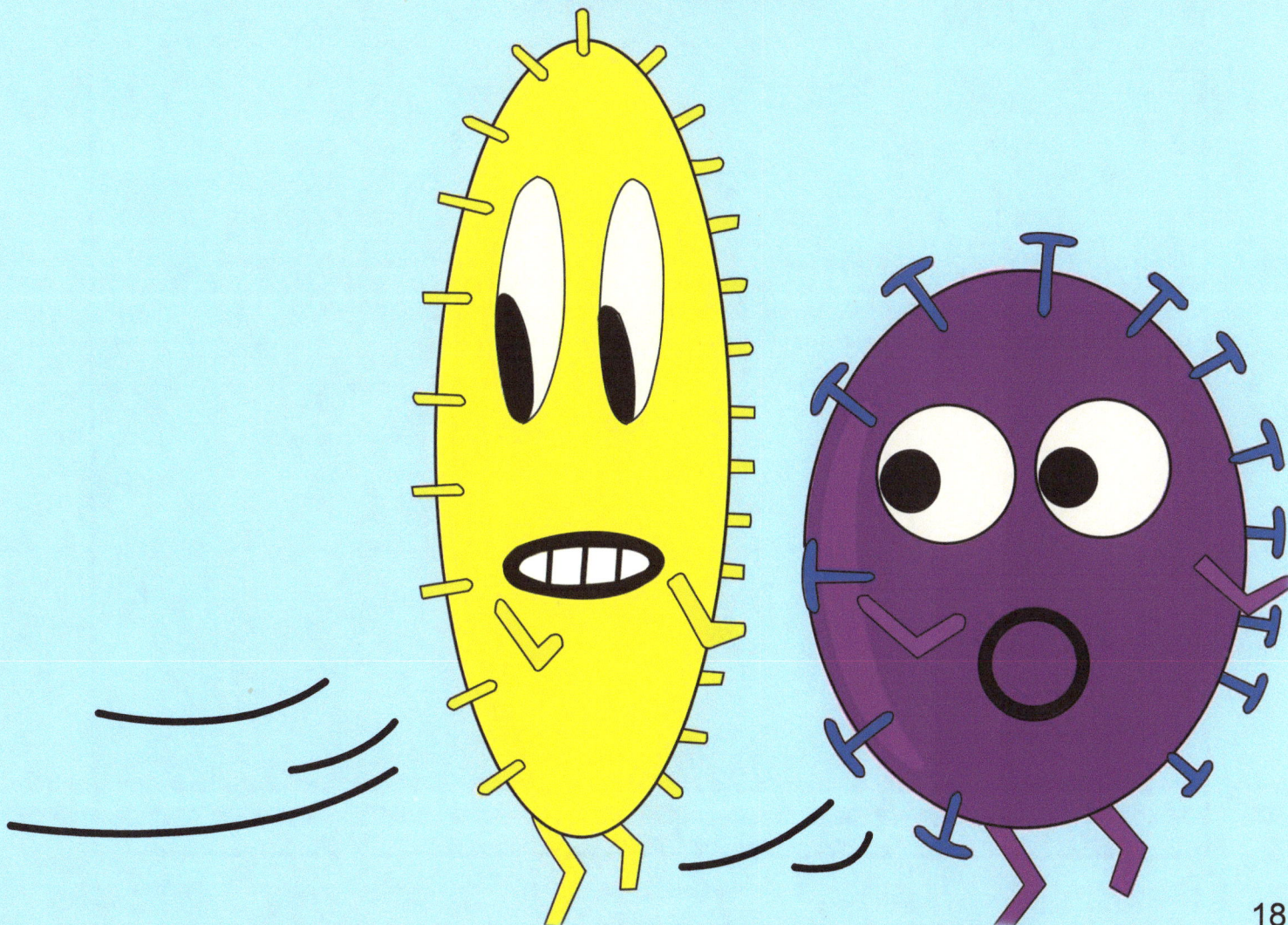

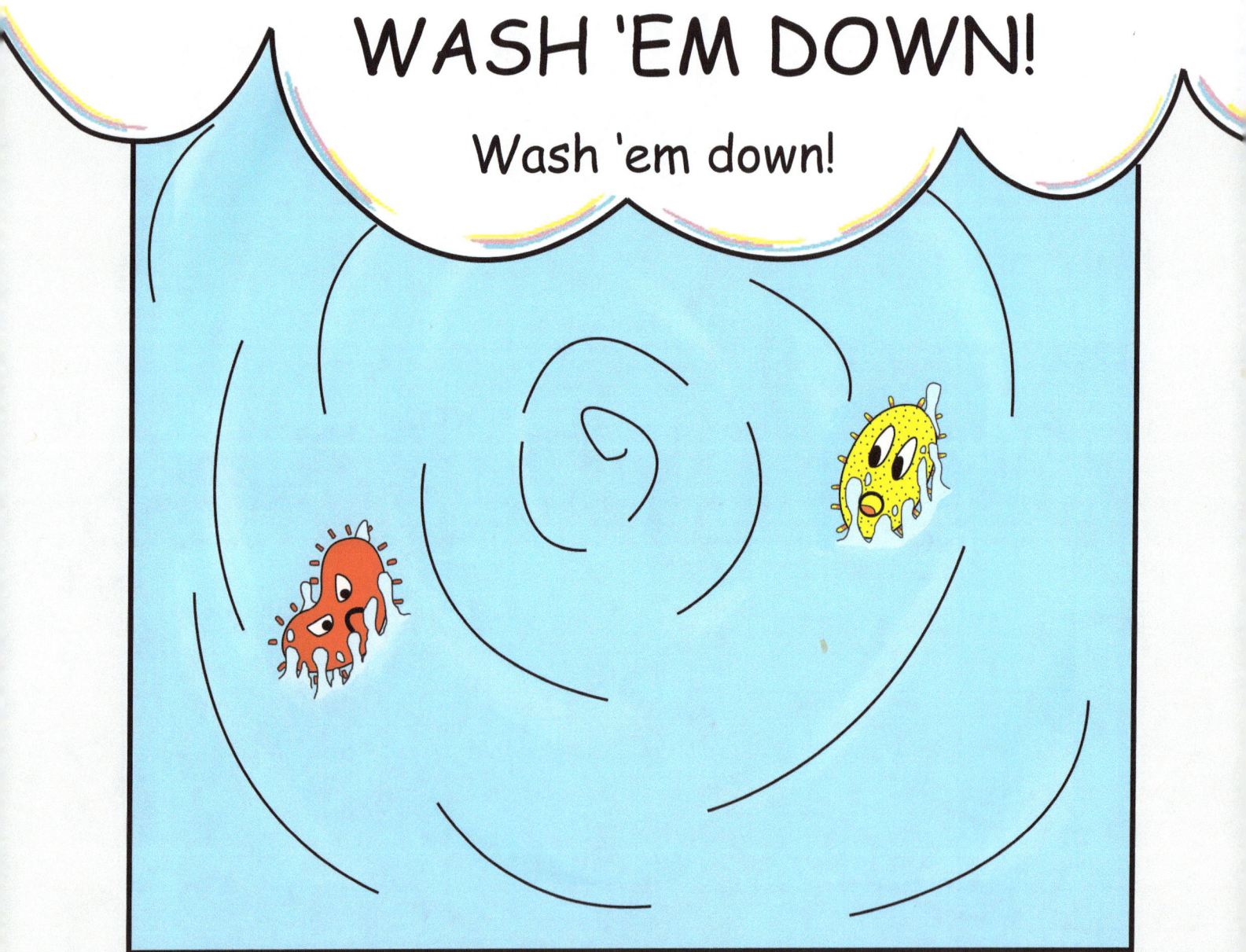

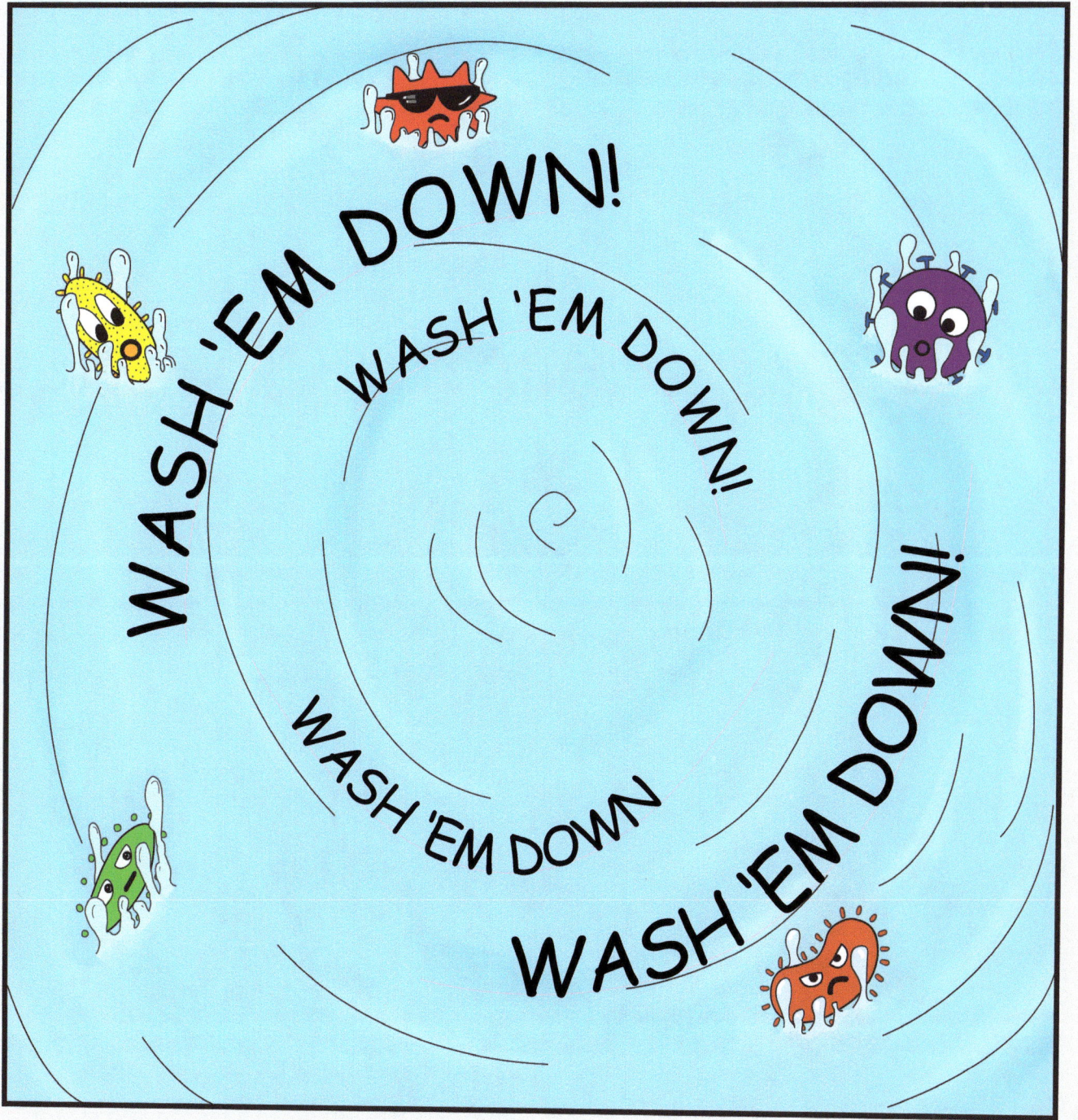

WASH 'EM DOWN!
WASH 'EM DOWN!
WASH 'EM DOWN
WASH 'EM DOWN!

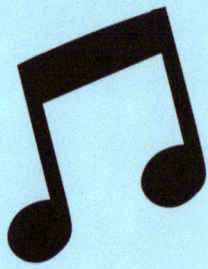

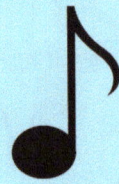

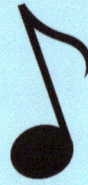

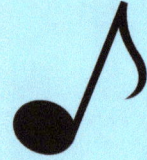

Check out these other Cool Cat songs!

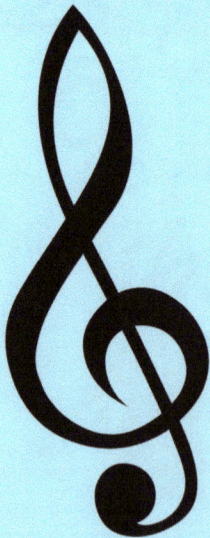

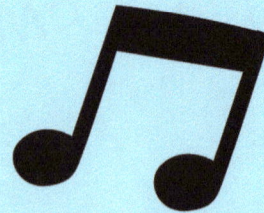

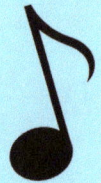

Swag Sentences

To the tune of "Calling My Phone" by Lil Tjjay ft. 6lack ©Columbia Records & Sony Music Entertainment

Rap-Along Here: https://www.youtube.com/watch?v=OCMnT8xPzog

Verse 1

We steady practicing sentences.

I done told you before that a sentence must have swag.

We know it's hurting because you think it's bad.

But our teacher is going to show us that we can brag,

About sentences having swag, having swag!

Chorus (2x)

Start with a capital letter.

Write the sentence neatly.

Put a space between our words.

Going to give it punctuation.

Start with a capital letter.

Write the sentence neatly.

Put a space between our words.

Going to give it punctuation.

Short Vowels

To the tune of "Astronaut in the Ocean" by Masked Wolf © Elektra Records

Rap-Along Here: https://www.youtube.com/watch?v=cKNbp4ZHtZc

Cool Cats Back

Tell me what you know about them vowels when you read.

A vowel is a letter you can say without your teeth.

When you are not using vowels, It's like not using lotion.

We about to show you how to put these vowels into motion.

(2x)

A E I O U (yeah yeah, yeah that's true).

A E I O U (short vowels, that's us).

Max has a black cat (a, a).

Ken yells right back (e, e).

Jill hit slick Rick (i, i).

Stop, drop, and roll in the sun (o, u).

One vowels, one word is usually short.

Sam ram had yams (Yes Mam).

Ted led red sled (Go head).

Kid hid pig wig (he did it).

Don't forget about the 'o' mop drop top.

Gus's cubs grubs on rugs (sho nuff).

That's the end of our vowel song.

That wasn't long.

Shout out to Masked Wolf and his song!

Words Have Syl-la-bles

To the tune of "Up" by Cardi B © Atlantic Records

Rap-Along Here: https://www.youtube.com/watch?v=wTsW6Ln6qHM

Once upon a time, I heard that syllables are the beat of words,

Coming straight from Cool Cats and Teacher T's World.

There's six syllable types:

Controlled r, consonant L E, VC silent e, Closed, Open, Vowel Team.

Hit em with that strategy,

Decoding words is easy!

Every syllable has a vowel in it

(I know that's right).

Closed syllables is closed by a consonant.

Open syllables end with a long vowel sound.

Closed syllables is closed by a consonant.

Open syllables end with a long vowel sound.

Like stuff, most, dog, peck, fun (then its closed).

If it's go, he, she, acorn, no, (then its open).

If it's junk (then its closed).

If it's Hi (then its open).

If it's we, cry bed (its open and closed).

Problems Up

To the tune of "Bottoms Up" by Trey Songz ft Nicki Minaj © Atlantic Records

Rap-Along Here: https://www.youtube.com/watch?v=_HvQFGfv2BI

Problems up, Problems up (up).

Throw your hands up!

Tell 'em it's a problem,

We about to blow these problems up!

Problems up, Problems up (up).

Throw your hands up!

Tell 'em it's a problem,

We about to blow these problems up!

Problems up, Problems up (up).

You know what we need.

We're doing our math and we're keeping it
clean.

Problems up, Problems up (up)

Throw your hands up!

Tell 'em it's a problem,

We about to blow these problems up!

Do the Floss (4x)

Hit the shoot (4x)

Now Milly Rock, aye (4x)

Orange Justice (4x)

Hit the Woah (4x)

Let me see you do the mop, aye (4x)

Hit the Dab (4x)

Now superman, aye (4x)

Throw them L's up (4x)

Let's kill this math (4x)

Take a seat (2x)

Take a load off your feet

Take a seat (2x)

Take a load off your feet

Fact Families

To the tune of "Bodak Yellow" by Cardi B © Atlantic Records

Rap-Along Here: https://www.youtube.com/watch?v=pxLR__IRaS0

Say, little children,

You can add and subtract.

If you wanted to

Using fact families

Is one way that we choose to do.

There are three numbers in a family that we must include,

And we're learning how to add and subtract so we are comfortable.

Look

We have to put them into four equations,

Two addition and two subtraction.

If you see that you can't do it,

Then you must not give up dude.

I'm a teacher and you're a cool cat,

And we're making Math cool!

Adjectives

To the tune of "Savage" by Megan Thee Stallion © 1501 Certified Entertainment and 300 Entertainment

Rap-Along Here: https://www.youtube.com/watch?v=K7n9tL9uNRs

Teacher T's here come and learn with me.

I'm going to teach you how to describe nouns properly.

A noun is a person, place, or thing.

After this you will describe nouns easily.

I'm an adjective a noun describer.

If you use me then your sentence will be fire.

Parts of a speech can be descriptive and fancy.

This an easy lesson you will quickly understand it. (ah)

Adjectives can help you with sen-ten-ces, truly.

They can be color words that describe you and me.

I can go before or after a noun so you see,

This is Teacher T and the Cool Cats.

Chorus

I'm an adjective:

Smart, funny, active

Busy, little, attractive

Witty, magnificent, outstanding

Outstanding, we're adjectives (2x)

Outstanding!

I joined Tik Tok by chance.

I wanna take this time to thank all my fans.

Teacher T is here, and I hope you understand.

If you wanna hear some real adjectives, baby here's your chance!

I say these beautiful girls and handsome boys are Cool Cats we became.

Camilla up in this thang, let's add fuel this flame.

I been killing it in the classroom with my gang, gang, gang, gang.

If you ain't been rocking with me then you should want to hop on this wave.

Continue to keep me hyped and supply us with those wipes.

And I promise to give it my all and that will definitely suffice.

I'm a boss, I'm a teacher, and I'll find a way to reach ya.

Remember adjectives are just noun describers that you can decipher.

Chorus (2x)

27

Possessive Nouns

To the tune of "Meant to Be" by Bebe Rexha © Warner Records

Rap-Along Here: https://www.youtube.com/watch?v=xQKfgz2KiZQ

Verse 1

We already know a lot about nouns.
Possessive nouns always show ownership.
With apostrophe 's' at the end,
let's get on down right here with this skill.

These nouns must be written in entirety.
We got nothing but time.
Then you add the possessive ending.
See, you are going to do just fine.

Chorus

Possessive nouns belong to me, belong to me,
Possessive nouns belong to me
(x2)

So, write em down with me, down with me.
See where this thing goes.
Possessive nouns belong to me, belong to me,
possessive nouns belong to me.

Verse 2

Remember nouns are a person, place, or thing
like Teacher T, Walmart, or a string.
Possessive nouns is about apostrophe.
Ain't gunna lie, it's going to be tricky.

To make the singular noun possessive,
Add an apostrophe and add an 's'.
To make the plural noun possessive,
Just go on and add the apostrophe.

Chorus (x2)

So, write em down with me, down with me
See where this thing goes.
Possessive nouns belong to me, belong to me,
possessive nouns belong to me.
So, write em down with me, down with me
See where this thing goes.
Possessive nouns belong to me, belong to me,
possessive nouns belong to me.

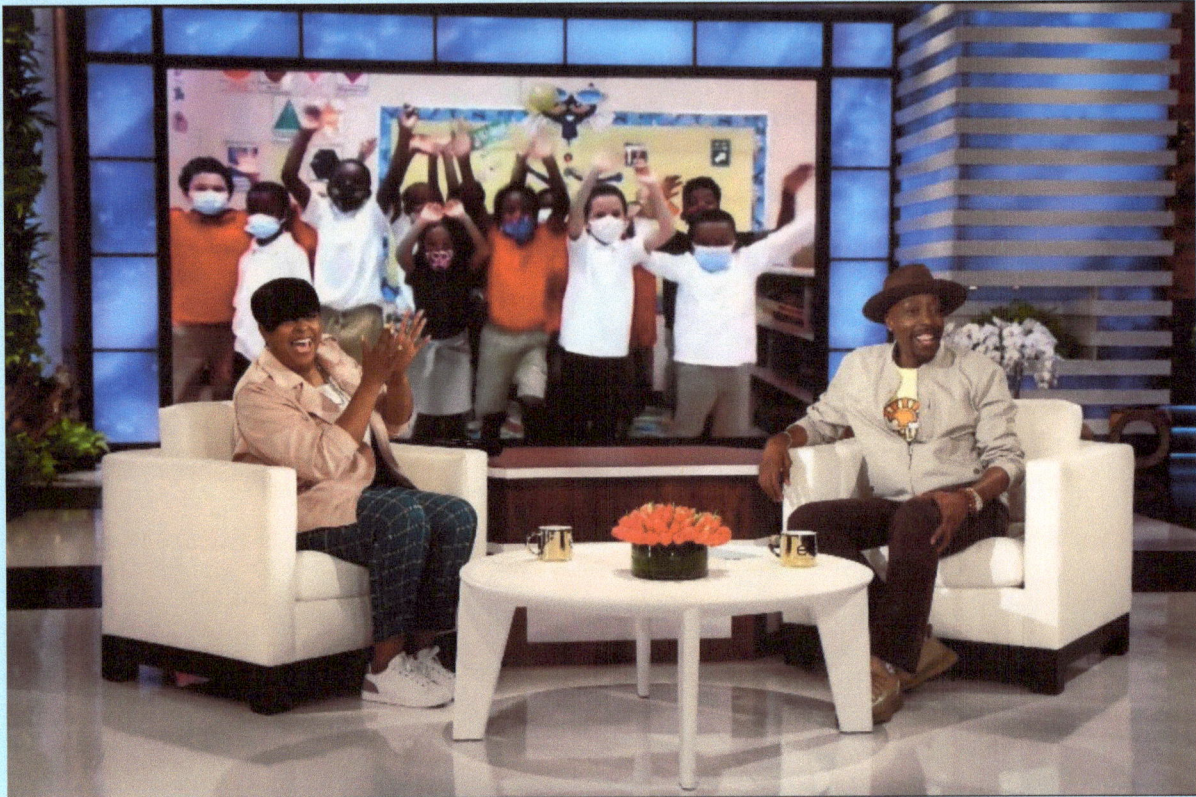

Tamika Mitchell-Wilcher and her Cool Cats on The Ellen Show with host, Arsenio Hall.

Acknowledgements

I am eternally grateful for all of my **"Cool Cats"** that I have had the
opportunity to stand before and lead. Thank you for being my inspiration and
entering the classroom ready to learn each day.
I love you all so very much!

Special thanks goes to the best bosses a girl could ask for,
Mrs. Donna B. Johnson and **Ms. Vicki Hicks.**
You both have always believed in me and allowed my creative juices to flow
inside of my classroom. You both are definitely "My Faves"!
I love you both to pieces.

To my husband, **Willie L. Wilcher,**
and my kids (**Markya, Xzavier, and Ma'Qell**),
thank you all for your continuous support and having my back.
I love you all to life!

I also want to thank my father-in-law, **Willie L. Wilcher, Sr.** for pushing me to
finish this project in a timely manner.
Your words and wisdom have brought me through so much.
You rock and I love you!

Last but not least, to my editor, **Ashley Dowell**, thank you for all of your ideas
and input. I love you, your honesty and your kind spirit. Thank you for all that
you have done.